DIABETIC CAKE RECIPES COOKBOOK

Sugar Free Cakes for Diabetics

LIAM LUXE

INTRODUCTION

This cookbook has been carefully crafted to cater to the needs of individuals living with diabetes while still allowing them to enjoy the delectable pleasure of cakes. Diabetes management often requires a balanced diet with limited sugar and carbohydrates, which can make enjoying sweet treats seem challenging. However, with the right ingredients and techniques, it's possible to create delicious cakes that won't compromise your blood sugar levels.

In this cookbook, we aim to provide a diverse array of diabetic-friendly cake recipes, ranging from flourless cakes and low-sugar sponge cakes to fruit-based delights and indulgent chocolate creations. Each recipe has been thoughtfully developed, keeping in mind the dietary requirements and nutritional considerations for individuals with diabetes.

Chaptered Delights: Our cookbook comprises several chapters, each dedicated to a specific type of diabetic cake. You'll find recipes for flourless cakes that are rich and luscious without the need for traditional flour. For those who prefer classic sponge cakes, we have curated low-sugar alternatives that retain all the flavor and charm without the sugar spike. If you crave fruity goodness, our fruit-based cake recipes will tantalize your taste buds with natural sweetness.

Indulgent Chocolate Creations: Chocoholics need not worry, as we have a dedicated chapter that features mouthwatering chocolate cakes, expertly crafted to satisfy your cocoa cravings without compromising your health. We've utilized ingredients that add depth and richness to these creations, ensuring that you won't miss the sugar-laden versions.

Special Occasion Cakes and More: Life's special moments call for exceptional cakes. Our collection includes unique recipes for special occasions that will impress guests and delight your loved ones. From sugar-free Red Velvet Cake to a show-stopping Pistachio Rosewater Celebration Cake, these recipes offer a taste of luxury without the guilt.

Beyond Sweet: Savory and Savory-Sweet Cakes: In addition to sweet cakes, we've explored the realm of savory and savory-sweet creations that can serve as delightful snacks or accompaniments to meals. These cakes showcase the versatility of diabetic-friendly baking, proving that you can enjoy cake-like treats even in your savory moments.

Frostings and Glazes: A cake is not complete without the perfect finishing touch. Our cookbook includes a range of frosting and glaze recipes, designed to complement the cakes while maintaining diabetic-friendly standards. These options provide the perfect balance of sweetness and flavor enhancement.

We hope this cookbook inspires you to embark on a delightful journey of baking and savoring delicious diabetic-friendly cakes. Always remember to consult your healthcare provider or a nutritionist to personalize your dietary choices based on your specific health needs. Let this book be your trusted companion in creating treats that are both indulgent and nourishing, allowing you to savor every bite with peace of mind. Happy baking!

CONTENTS

FLOURLESS CAKE RECIPES

Welcome to the delectable world of flourless cake recipes, where we explore the art of creating sumptuous cakes without traditional wheat flour. These delightful treats are not only perfect for individuals with gluten sensitivities but also a fantastic option for those looking to reduce their carbohydrate intake without compromising on taste or texture.

In this chapter, we have carefully curated a selection of flourless cakes that embrace alternative flours and ingredients, offering a delightful array of flavors and culinary experiences. Each recipe has been thoughtfully crafted to provide a moist and tender crumb, ensuring that you won't miss the presence of wheat flour in the slightest.

Indulge in the richness of our Decadent Chocolate Avocado Cake, where the creamy goodness of avocado combines harmoniously with the intensity of dark chocolate. Or perhaps you prefer a citrusy delight, in which case the Zesty Lemon Almond Cake will tantalize your taste buds with its refreshing and aromatic essence.

For those who relish the classic combination of fruits and nuts, our Moist Carrot Walnut Cake provides a wholesome and delightful experience. The natural sweetness of carrots and the earthiness of walnuts create a harmonious marriage of flavors that are both satisfying and nourishing.

Whether you're a seasoned baker or a newcomer to the world of flourless cakes, this chapter has something to offer everyone.

1.1 Decadent Chocolate Avocado Cake

Ingredients:

- 2 ripe avocados, pitted and peeled
- 200g dark chocolate (70% cocoa or higher), chopped
- 1/2 cup unsweetened cocoa powder
- 1/2 cup almond flour
- 1 teaspoon baking powder
- 1/4 teaspoon salt
- 3 large eggs
- 1/2 cup granulated sugar substitute (e.g., erythritol, stevia)
- 1 teaspoon vanilla extract
- Optional: 1/4 cup chopped walnuts or pecans for added texture and flavor

Instructions:

1. Preheat your oven to 350°F (175°C). Grease an 8-inch round cake pan and line the bottom with parchment paper for easy removal.

2. In a microwave-safe bowl, melt the dark chocolate in 30-second intervals, stirring in between, until smooth. Set aside to cool slightly.

3. In a blender or food processor, combine the ripe avocados and melted chocolate. Blend until smooth and creamy.

4. In a separate mixing bowl, whisk together the unsweetened cocoa powder, almond flour, baking powder, and salt until well combined.

5. In a large mixing bowl, beat the eggs and sugar substitute until light and fluffy. Stir in the avocado-chocolate mixture and

vanilla extract until fully incorporated.

6. Gradually add the dry ingredients to the wet ingredients and mix until you have a smooth batter. If using nuts, fold them into the batter.

7. Pour the batter into the prepared cake pan and smooth the top with a spatula.

8. Bake in the preheated oven for approximately 25-30 minutes or until a toothpick inserted into the center comes out with a few moist crumbs (not wet batter).

9. Remove the cake from the oven and let it cool in the pan for 10 minutes. Then, carefully transfer it to a wire rack to cool completely.

10. Once cooled, you can dust the cake with a little cocoa powder or top it with your favorite glaze (sugar-free glaze if preferred) for added indulgence.

Nutritional Information (Approximate, per serving):

- Calories: 220 kcal
- Total Fat: 16g
    - Saturated Fat: 6g
- Cholesterol: 60mg
- Sodium: 90mg
- Total Carbohydrates: 18g
    - Dietary Fiber: 7g
    - Sugars: 1g
- Protein: 6g

Please note that the nutritional information provided is an estimate and may vary based on the specific ingredients and brands used. Always double-check the labels of the ingredients you use to calculate the most accurate nutritional information for your cake.

Enjoy your Decadent Chocolate Avocado Cake as a delightful and healthier alternative to traditional chocolate cakes!

1.2 Zesty Lemon Almond Cake

The combination of almond flour and ground almonds in this recipe not only adds a delectable texture but also imparts a delightful nuttiness that perfectly complements the zesty lemon flavor. The absence of traditional flour makes this cake gluten-free and suitable for those with gluten sensitivities.

This cake is not overly sweet, allowing the natural citrus flavors to shine through. However, feel free to adjust the sweetness to your preference by using your favorite sugar substitute. A drizzle of lemon glaze or a light dusting of powdered sugar can add an elegant finish to this already delightful treat.

Bake this Zesty Lemon Almond Cake for brunch gatherings, afternoon tea, or any time you crave a refreshing and indulgent treat. Its light, moist crumb and captivating lemon flavor make it a versatile and delightful addition to your repertoire of flourless cake recipes.

Ingredients:

- 1 cup almond flour
- 1/2 cup ground almonds (almond meal)
- 1 teaspoon baking powder
- 1/4 teaspoon salt
- 3 large eggs
- 1/2 cup granulated sugar substitute (e.g., erythritol, stevia)
- Zest of 2 lemons (about 2 tablespoons)
- 1/4 cup fresh lemon juice
- 1/3 cup unsweetened applesauce
- 1 teaspoon pure vanilla extract

Optional Lemon Glaze:

- 1/2 cup powdered sugar substitute (e.g., powdered erythritol)
- 2 tablespoons fresh lemon juice

- Zest of 1 lemon (optional, for garnish)

Instructions:

1. Preheat your oven to 350°F (175°C). Grease an 8-inch round cake pan and line the bottom with parchment paper.

2. In a mixing bowl, whisk together the almond flour, ground almonds, baking powder, and salt until well combined.

3. In a separate large mixing bowl, beat the eggs and sugar substitute until light and fluffy. Stir in the lemon zest, lemon juice, unsweetened applesauce, and vanilla extract.

4. Gradually add the dry ingredients to the wet ingredients and mix until you have a smooth batter.

5. Pour the batter into the prepared cake pan and smooth the top with a spatula.

6. Bake in the preheated oven for approximately 25-30 minutes or until a toothpick inserted into the center comes out with a few moist crumbs.

7. While the cake is baking, prepare the optional lemon glaze by whisking together the powdered sugar substitute and fresh lemon juice until smooth.

8. Remove the cake from the oven and let it cool in the pan for 10 minutes. Then, carefully transfer it to a wire rack to cool completely.

9. Once the cake is cooled, drizzle the lemon glaze over the top, and if desired, sprinkle with additional lemon zest for a burst of color and flavor.

Nutritional Information (Approximate, per serving, without glaze):

- Calories: 180 kcal
- Total Fat: 13g
  - Saturated Fat: 1g
- Cholesterol: 55mg

- Sodium: 130mg

- Total Carbohydrates: 9g

  - Dietary Fiber: 3g

  - Sugars: 1g

- Protein: 7g

Enjoy the refreshing and delightful flavors of our Zesty Lemon Almond Cake, a gluten-free treat that will add a touch of sunshine to your day. Serve it as a lovely dessert or alongside your favorite cup of tea for a delightful afternoon indulgence.

1.3 Moist Carrot Walnut Cake

This flourless wonder combines the natural sweetness of carrots, the earthy crunch of walnuts, and a touch of warm spices to create a moist and satisfying treat that is both comforting and nourishing.

Carrots take center stage in this recipe, providing natural sweetness, moisture, and a boost of nutrients, including beta-carotene, vitamin A, and fiber. The combination of almond flour and ground walnuts lends a rich, nutty depth to the cake, creating a delightful contrast of textures with every bite.

In addition to being flourless, this cake is lightly sweetened with your choice of sugar substitute, making it an excellent option for those looking to reduce their sugar intake while still enjoying a delectable dessert.

The aromatic spices of cinnamon and nutmeg infuse the cake with cozy warmth, reminiscent of a homemade carrot cake straight from the oven. Whether you're serving it for dessert or as a special treat for breakfast or brunch, this Moist Carrot Walnut Cake is sure to become a beloved favorite.

Ingredients:

- 1 cup almond flour

- 1/2 cup ground walnuts (walnut meal)

- 1 teaspoon baking powder

- 1/2 teaspoon ground cinnamon
- 1/4 teaspoon ground nutmeg
- 1/4 teaspoon salt
- 3 large eggs
- 1/2 cup granulated sugar substitute (e.g., erythritol, stevia)
- 1/3 cup unsweetened applesauce
- 1 teaspoon pure vanilla extract
- 1 1/2 cups grated carrots (about 2-3 medium-sized carrots)
- 1/2 cup chopped walnuts (for added texture and garnish)

Optional Cream Cheese Frosting:

- 4 ounces cream cheese (full-fat), softened
- 2 tablespoons powdered sugar substitute (e.g., powdered erythritol)
- 1/2 teaspoon pure vanilla extract

Instructions:

1. Preheat your oven to 350°F (175°C). Grease an 8-inch round cake pan and line the bottom with parchment paper.

2. In a mixing bowl, whisk together the almond flour, ground walnuts, baking powder, ground cinnamon, ground nutmeg, and salt until well combined.

3. In a separate large mixing bowl, beat the eggs and sugar substitute until light and fluffy. Stir in the unsweetened applesauce and pure vanilla extract.

4. Gradually add the dry ingredients to the wet ingredients and mix until you have a smooth batter.

5. Fold in the grated carrots and chopped walnuts, distributing them evenly throughout the batter.

6. Pour the batter into the prepared cake pan and smooth the top with a spatula.

7. Bake in the preheated oven for approximately 30-35 minutes or until a toothpick inserted into the center comes out clean.

8. Remove the cake from the oven and let it cool in the pan for 10 minutes. Then, carefully transfer it to a wire rack to cool completely.

Optional Cream Cheese Frosting:

1. In a mixing bowl, beat the softened cream cheese until smooth.

2. Add the powdered sugar substitute and pure vanilla extract to the cream cheese and continue to beat until well combined.

3. Once the cake is completely cooled, spread the cream cheese frosting over the top of the cake.

4. Garnish with additional chopped walnuts, if desired, for added texture and visual appeal.

Nutritional Information (Approximate, per serving, without frosting):

- Calories: 200 kcal
- Total Fat: 16g
  - Saturated Fat: 3g
- Cholesterol: 55mg
- Sodium: 95mg
- Total Carbohydrates: 9g
  - Dietary Fiber: 3g
  - Sugars: 2g
- Protein: 7g

LOW-SUGAR SPONGE CAKES

Welcome to the delightful world of Low-Sugar Sponge Cakes, where we reimagine classic sponge cake recipes with a healthy twist. In this chapter, we present a collection of light and airy sponge cakes that are thoughtfully crafted to be lower in sugar without compromising on taste or texture.

Sponge cakes are beloved for their soft and tender crumb, making them a perfect canvas for various flavors and fillings. We've carefully designed these recipes to be lower in sugar content, allowing you to enjoy the simple pleasure of a moist and delicious cake without the worry of a sugar overload.

2.1 Classic Victoria Sponge Cake (Sugar-Free)

The beauty of a Victoria Sponge lies in its simplicity—a delicate sponge cake layered with luscious fillings, making it the epitome of refined indulgence. In our sugar-free adaptation, we've replaced the conventional sugar with a suitable sugar substitute, ensuring that you can enjoy this classic delicacy without compromising your dietary goals.

The secret to the sponge's light and airy texture lies in the perfect balance of ingredients. Our low-sugar version utilizes a combination of almond flour and a touch of cornstarch, creating a sponge that is not only gluten-free but also lower in carbohydrates.

To maintain the signature Victoria Sponge charm, we've crafted a delightful filling using sugar-free fruit preserves or fresh berries, layered with a dollop of unsweetened whipped cream or a sugar substitute-based cream. The result is a delightful contrast of textures and flavors that evoke memories of afternoon gatherings and cherished moments with loved ones.

Whether you're hosting a tea party or simply treating yourself to an afternoon indulgence, our Classic Victoria Sponge Cake (Sugar-Free) is sure to impress. With its light and tender crumb, paired with the gentle sweetness of the filling, this cake is a testament to the art of baking with both taste and health in mind.

Ingredients:

- 1 cup almond flour
- 1/4 cup cornstarch
- 1 teaspoon baking powder
- 1/4 teaspoon salt
- 4 large eggs, at room temperature
- 1/2 cup granulated sugar substitute (e.g., erythritol, stevia)
- 1 teaspoon pure vanilla extract
- 1/2 cup sugar-free fruit preserves or fresh berries (e.g., raspberry, strawberry)
- 1 cup unsweetened whipped cream or sugar substitute-based cream

Instructions:

1. Preheat your oven to 350°F (175°C). Grease two 8-inch round cake pans and line the bottoms with parchment paper.

2. In a mixing bowl, whisk together the almond flour, cornstarch, baking powder, and salt until well combined.

3. In a separate large mixing bowl, beat the eggs and sugar substitute until pale and fluffy. Stir in the pure vanilla extract.

4. Gradually fold the dry ingredients into the egg mixture until

you have a smooth batter.

5. Divide the batter evenly between the prepared cake pans and smooth the tops with a spatula.

6. Bake in the preheated oven for approximately 20-25 minutes or until the cakes are golden brown and a toothpick inserted into the center comes out clean.

7. Remove the cakes from the oven and let them cool in the pans for 10 minutes. Then, carefully transfer them to a wire rack to cool completely.

8. Once the cakes are completely cooled, spread the sugar-free fruit preserves or fresh berries on one cake layer.

9. On the other cake layer, spread the unsweetened whipped cream or sugar substitute-based cream.

10. Carefully place the cream-topped layer on the fruit preserves layer, creating a delightful sandwich.

11. Dust the top of the cake with a sprinkle of powdered sugar substitute or decorate with additional fresh berries, if desired.

Nutritional Information (Approximate, per serving):

- Calories: 220 kcal
- Total Fat: 18g
    - Saturated Fat: 6g
- Cholesterol: 90mg
- Sodium: 150mg
- Total Carbohydrates: 9g
    - Dietary Fiber: 2g
    - Sugars: 1g
- Protein: 6g

2.2 Raspberry and Vanilla Yogurt Cake

The star of this cake is the vibrant and juicy raspberries that are dotted throughout the moist sponge. These antioxidant-rich berries add a burst of color and a delightful tangy sweetness to each slice.

To create a moist and tender crumb, we've incorporated yogurt into the batter. The yogurt not only adds a subtle tang but also contributes to the cake's lightness, making it a delightful treat to enjoy any time of day.

For the perfect balance of sweetness without excessive sugar, we've opted for a sugar substitute or a minimal amount of natural sweeteners like honey or maple syrup. The result is a delightful cake that satisfies your sweet tooth while being kind to your health.

Whether you're hosting a brunch or celebrating a special occasion, our Raspberry and Vanilla Yogurt Cake is a delightful addition to your dessert repertoire. Serve it with a dollop of lightly sweetened whipped cream and an extra scattering of fresh raspberries for an impressive presentation.

Ingredients:

- 1 cup almond flour

- 1/4 cup cornstarch or coconut flour

- 1 teaspoon baking powder

- 1/4 teaspoon salt

- 4 large eggs, at room temperature

- 1/3 cup granulated sugar substitute or natural sweetener (e.g., honey, maple syrup)

- 1/2 cup plain Greek yogurt

- 1 teaspoon pure vanilla extract

- 1 cup fresh raspberries, plus extra for garnish

- Optional: Lightly sweetened whipped cream for serving

Instructions:

1. Preheat your oven to 350°F (175°C). Grease an 8-inch round cake pan and line the bottom with parchment paper.

2. In a mixing bowl, whisk together the almond flour, cornstarch or coconut flour, baking powder, and salt until well combined.

3. In a separate large mixing bowl, beat the eggs and sugar substitute or natural sweetener until pale and fluffy. Stir in the plain Greek yogurt and pure vanilla extract.

4. Gradually fold the dry ingredients into the egg-yogurt mixture until you have a smooth batter.

5. Gently fold in the fresh raspberries, being careful not to crush them.

6. Pour the batter into the prepared cake pan and smooth the top with a spatula.

7. Bake in the preheated oven for approximately 25-30 minutes or until the cake is golden brown and a toothpick inserted into the center comes out clean.

8. Remove the cake from the oven and let it cool in the pan for 10 minutes. Then, carefully transfer it to a wire rack to cool completely.

9. Once the cake is completely cooled, serve it with a dollop of lightly sweetened whipped cream and an extra scattering of fresh raspberries for a delightful and visually stunning presentation.

Nutritional Information (Approximate, per serving):

- Calories: 180 kcal
- Total Fat: 14g
  - Saturated Fat: 3g
- Cholesterol: 70mg
- Sodium: 140mg
- Total Carbohydrates: 8g
  - Dietary Fiber: 2g
  - Sugars: 1g
- Protein: 7g

2.3 Spiced Apple Cinnamon Cake

The star of this cake is the tender and juicy apples, which infuse the sponge with their delicate sweetness. As they bake, the apples release their delicious flavors, creating pockets of delightful fruitiness in every slice.

To capture the essence of autumn, we've artfully combined warm spices such as cinnamon, nutmeg, and cloves, enhancing the cake with their comforting and aromatic charm. The subtle balance of these spices elevates the cake's flavor profile, making it a truly indulgent experience.

For a mindful and balanced sweetness, we've opted for a sugar substitute or a modest amount of natural sweeteners like honey or maple syrup. The result is a cake that beautifully captures the essence of apple season without overwhelming your taste buds with excessive sugar.

Our Spiced Apple Cinnamon Cake is perfect for serving on cozy evenings, paired with a warm cup of tea or coffee. It also makes a delightful addition to autumn gatherings, filling the air with the inviting aroma of baked apples and spices.

Ingredients:

- 1 cup almond flour
- 1/4 cup coconut flour
- 1 teaspoon baking powder
- 1/2 teaspoon ground cinnamon
- 1/4 teaspoon ground nutmeg
- 1/8 teaspoon ground cloves
- 1/4 teaspoon salt
- 4 large eggs, at room temperature
- 1/3 cup granulated sugar substitute or natural sweetener (e.g., honey, maple syrup)
- 1/2 cup unsweetened applesauce

- 1 teaspoon pure vanilla extract

- 1 1/2 cups peeled and diced apples (about 2 medium-sized apples)

- Optional: Additional apple slices for garnish

Instructions:

1. Preheat your oven to 350°F (175°C). Grease an 8-inch round cake pan and line the bottom with parchment paper.

2. In a mixing bowl, whisk together the almond flour, coconut flour, baking powder, ground cinnamon, ground nutmeg, ground cloves, and salt until well combined.

3. In a separate large mixing bowl, beat the eggs and sugar substitute or natural sweetener until pale and fluffy. Stir in the unsweetened applesauce and pure vanilla extract.

4. Gradually fold the dry ingredients into the egg-applesauce mixture until you have a smooth batter.

5. Gently fold in the peeled and diced apples, distributing them evenly throughout the batter.

6. Pour the batter into the prepared cake pan and smooth the top with a spatula.

7. If desired, arrange a few apple slices on top of the batter for an elegant garnish.

8. Bake in the preheated oven for approximately 30-35 minutes or until the cake is golden brown and a toothpick inserted into the center comes out clean.

9. Remove the cake from the oven and let it cool in the pan for 10 minutes. Then, carefully transfer it to a wire rack to cool completely.

10. Serve the Spiced Apple Cinnamon Cake as a delightful dessert or enjoy it alongside your favorite cup of warm beverage for a cozy autumn treat.

Nutritional Information (Approximate, per serving):

- Calories: 190 kcal

- Total Fat: 15g
  - Saturated Fat: 3g
- Cholesterol: 70mg
- Sodium: 140mg
- Total Carbohydrates: 8g
  - Dietary Fiber: 3g
  - Sugars: 2g
- Protein: 7g

NUTRITIOUS FRUIT-BASED CAKES

Fruits are nature's sweet gift, bursting with flavors and vibrant colors that add a touch of magic to any dessert. We've carefully crafted these fruit-based cakes to showcase the best of seasonal produce, allowing you to celebrate the joys of each fruit's peak freshness.

From the succulent sweetness of berries and peaches to the tropical allure of mangoes and pineapples, each recipe features a different fruit as the star ingredient. Our goal is to elevate the natural flavors of fruits while ensuring that the cakes remain balanced and nutrient-rich.

To enhance the nutritional profile of these cakes, we've opted for alternative flours and sugar substitutes that reduce refined carbohydrates without compromising on taste or texture. You'll find the use of almond flour, coconut flour, or whole wheat flour, along with the incorporation of sugar substitutes like stevia, erythritol, or maple syrup.

Each cake is thoughtfully designed to provide you with a guilt-free indulgence, making them suitable for those with dietary restrictions or health-conscious individuals looking to embrace the benefits of fruit-based desserts.

3.1 Mixed Berry Chia Seed Cake

Berries, with their natural sweetness and stunning colors, take center stage in this recipe. From plump blueberries to juicy strawberries and tangy raspberries, each bite offers a burst of fruity goodness. Packed with antioxidants, vitamins, and fiber, the mixed berries not only lend their delightful flavors but also infuse the cake with a touch of natural vibrancy.

Chia seeds, the nutrient-packed superfood, play a vital role in elevating this cake's nutritional profile. These tiny powerhouses are rich in omega-3 fatty acids, protein, and fiber, providing a delightful crunch and enhancing the cake's satiety factor.

Our Mixed Berry Chia Seed Cake is crafted with a blend of alternative flours and sugar substitutes, keeping refined carbohydrates at bay. The combination of almond flour, coconut flour, or whole wheat flour offers a wholesome foundation, while sugar substitutes like stevia or erythritol add a delicate sweetness that complements the natural sweetness of the berries.

Perfect for brunch gatherings, afternoon teas, or any time you crave a nourishing dessert, this cake showcases the beauty of simplicity while delivering a burst of flavors that will leave you craving for more.

Ingredients:

- 1 cup almond flour
- 1/4 cup coconut flour
- 1/4 cup chia seeds
- 1 teaspoon baking powder
- 1/4 teaspoon salt
- 4 large eggs, at room temperature
- 1/3 cup granulated sugar substitute (e.g., stevia, erythritol)
- 1/2 cup unsweetened applesauce or mashed ripe banana
- 1 teaspoon pure vanilla extract

- 1 cup mixed berries (blueberries, strawberries, raspberries)
- Optional: Fresh berries for garnish

Instructions:

1. Preheat your oven to 350°F (175°C). Grease an 8-inch round cake pan and line the bottom with parchment paper.

2. In a mixing bowl, whisk together the almond flour, coconut flour, chia seeds, baking powder, and salt until well combined.

3. In a separate large mixing bowl, beat the eggs and sugar substitute until pale and fluffy. Stir in the unsweetened applesauce or mashed ripe banana and pure vanilla extract.

4. Gradually fold the dry ingredients into the egg-applesauce mixture until you have a smooth batter.

5. Gently fold in the mixed berries, distributing them evenly throughout the batter.

6. Pour the batter into the prepared cake pan and smooth the top with a spatula.

7. If desired, arrange a few fresh berries on top of the batter for an elegant garnish.

8. Bake in the preheated oven for approximately 30-35 minutes or until the cake is golden brown and a toothpick inserted into the center comes out clean.

9. Remove the cake from the oven and let it cool in the pan for 10 minutes. Then, carefully transfer it to a wire rack to cool completely.

10. Serve the Mixed Berry Chia Seed Cake as a delightful dessert or as a nourishing afternoon treat.

Nutritional Information (Approximate, per serving):

- Calories: 180 kcal
- Total Fat: 13g
  - Saturated Fat: 2g
- Cholesterol: 70mg

- Sodium: 140mg
- Total Carbohydrates: 10g
  - Dietary Fiber: 5g
  - Sugars: 2g
- Protein: 7g

3.2 Sugarless Banana Walnut Cake

Ripe bananas are the star of this recipe, providing natural sweetness and moisture to the cake. The bananas not only create a delightful flavor profile but also add essential vitamins, minerals, and fiber to each slice.

To keep the cake sugarless, we rely on the sweetness of the ripe bananas and incorporate a sugar substitute to enhance the taste without overpowering the natural flavors. The result is a cake that is gentle on your blood sugar levels while delivering a delicious and satisfying experience.

Walnuts play a pivotal role in this cake, adding a delightful nutty flavor and a satisfying crunch. Packed with heart-healthy fats and essential nutrients, walnuts elevate the cake's nutritional value while adding a delightful texture to each bite.

Our Sugarless Banana Walnut Cake is crafted with alternative flours that reduce refined carbohydrates. Whether you choose almond flour, coconut flour, or a blend of both, the result is a cake that is gluten-free, low in carbs, and suitable for various dietary preferences.

Bake this cake for breakfast, dessert, or a wholesome snack, and savor the warmth and comfort of its flavors. Enjoy the delightful aroma of ripe bananas and toasted walnuts as they fill your kitchen with the essence of homemade goodness.

Ingredients:

- 1 cup almond flour or coconut flour (or a combination of both)
- 1 teaspoon baking powder
- 1/2 teaspoon ground cinnamon

- 1/4 teaspoon salt

- 4 large ripe bananas, mashed

- 4 large eggs, at room temperature

- 1/3 cup granulated sugar substitute (e.g., stevia, erythritol)

- 1/3 cup unsweetened applesauce or plain Greek yogurt

- 1 teaspoon pure vanilla extract

- 1/2 cup chopped walnuts, plus extra for garnish

Instructions:

1. Preheat your oven to 350°F (175°C). Grease an 8-inch round cake pan and line the bottom with parchment paper.

2. In a mixing bowl, whisk together the almond flour or coconut flour (or combination), baking powder, ground cinnamon, and salt until well combined.

3. In a separate large mixing bowl, beat the mashed bananas and eggs until well blended. Stir in the granulated sugar substitute, unsweetened applesauce or Greek yogurt, and pure vanilla extract.

4. Gradually fold the dry ingredients into the wet ingredients until you have a smooth batter.

5. Gently fold in the chopped walnuts, distributing them evenly throughout the batter.

6. Pour the batter into the prepared cake pan and smooth the top with a spatula.

7. If desired, sprinkle some additional chopped walnuts on top of the batter for added texture and visual appeal.

8. Bake in the preheated oven for approximately 30-35 minutes or until the cake is golden brown and a toothpick inserted into the center comes out clean.

9. Remove the cake from the oven and let it cool in the pan for 10 minutes. Then, carefully transfer it to a wire rack to cool completely.

10. Serve the Sugarless Banana Walnut Cake as a delightful breakfast treat, a satisfying dessert, or a nourishing snack.

Nutritional Information (Approximate, per serving):

- Calories: 200 kcal
- Total Fat: 15g
  - Saturated Fat: 2g
- Cholesterol: 70mg
- Sodium: 140mg
- Total Carbohydrates: 12g
  - Dietary Fiber: 4g
  - Sugars: 4g
- Protein: 7g

3.3 Plum and Oatmeal Crumble Cake

Plums, with their sweet-tart flavor, lend their juicy goodness to this cake, infusing each bite with a burst of fruity delight. The natural sweetness of ripe plums pairs beautifully with the subtle nuttiness of oats, creating a harmonious blend that is both comforting and indulgent.

Oatmeal takes center stage in the crumble topping, adding a delightful crunch that complements the softness of the cake. Oats are a source of complex carbohydrates and fiber, making this cake a wholesome option for those seeking a more nourishing dessert.

To keep this cake refined sugar-free, we utilize a sugar substitute or a modest amount of natural sweeteners like honey or maple syrup. This ensures that you can indulge in the delectable sweetness of this cake without compromising your health goals.

The combination of almond flour and alternative flours keeps this cake gluten-free and provides a light and tender crumb that enhances the overall eating experience.

Our Plum and Oatmeal Crumble Cake is perfect for showcasing the abundance of seasonal fruits and elevating your dessert table with a delightful and nutrient-rich treat.

Ingredients:

- 1 cup almond flour
- 1/4 cup coconut flour
- 1/4 cup rolled oats
- 1 teaspoon baking powder
- 1/4 teaspoon ground cinnamon
- 1/4 teaspoon salt
- 4 large eggs, at room temperature
- 1/3 cup granulated sugar substitute (e.g., stevia, erythritol) or natural sweetener (e.g., honey, maple syrup)
- 1/3 cup unsweetened applesauce or plain Greek yogurt
- 1 teaspoon pure vanilla extract
- 1 1/2 cups fresh plums, pitted and sliced
- 1/4 cup rolled oats (for the crumble topping)
- 2 tablespoons chopped almonds (for the crumble topping)
- 1 tablespoon unsalted butter or coconut oil, melted (for the crumble topping)
- Optional: Greek yogurt or vanilla ice cream for serving

Instructions:

1. Preheat your oven to 350°F (175°C). Grease an 8-inch round cake pan and line the bottom with parchment paper.

2. In a mixing bowl, whisk together the almond flour, coconut flour, rolled oats, baking powder, ground cinnamon, and salt until well combined.

3. In a separate large mixing bowl, beat the eggs and granulated sugar substitute or natural sweetener until pale and fluffy. Stir in the unsweetened applesauce or Greek yogurt and pure vanilla extract.

4. Gradually fold the dry ingredients into the egg-applesauce mixture until you have a smooth batter.

5. Pour the batter into the prepared cake pan and smooth the top with a spatula.

6. Arrange the sliced plums on top of the batter in a decorative pattern.

7. In a small bowl, mix together the rolled oats, chopped almonds, and melted butter or coconut oil to create the crumble topping.

8. Sprinkle the crumble topping evenly over the sliced plums.

9. Bake in the preheated oven for approximately 30-35 minutes or until the cake is golden brown and a toothpick inserted into the center comes out clean.

10. Remove the cake from the oven and let it cool in the pan for 10 minutes. Then, carefully transfer it to a wire rack to cool completely.

11. Serve the Plum and Oatmeal Crumble Cake with a dollop of Greek yogurt or a scoop of vanilla ice cream for a delightful dessert experience.

Nutritional Information (Approximate, per serving):

- Calories: 180 kcal
- Total Fat: 12g
  - Saturated Fat: 3g
- Cholesterol: 70mg
- Sodium: 140mg
- Total Carbohydrates: 14g
  - Dietary Fiber: 4g
  - Sugars: 6g
- Protein: 6g

CHOCOLATE DELIGHTS

Chocolate, with its velvety texture and captivating aroma, has a way of captivating our senses like no other. Whether you prefer the smoothness of milk chocolate, the intensity of dark chocolate, or the perfect balance of bittersweet cocoa, our collection of chocolate cakes has something to delight every chocoholic's palate.

We've carefully curated these recipes to balance the sheer pleasure of chocolate with mindful considerations of health and dietary needs. From flourless options to low-sugar adaptations, we've thoughtfully crafted each cake to ensure you can indulge in the bliss of chocolate without compromising your well-being.

4.1 Rich Dark Chocolate Beetroot Cake

Dark chocolate takes center stage in this cake, infusing every morsel with its bittersweet richness. The deep cocoa notes create a decadent canvas that complements the sweet and tender essence of beetroots.

Beetroots, the unexpected star of this recipe, bring a natural sweetness and moistness to the cake. Their vibrant crimson hue adds visual allure and promises a delightful adventure for your palate.

To enhance the nutritional profile and maintain the rich texture of this cake, we've chosen a blend of alternative flours, such as almond flour or coconut flour. The result is a gluten-free delight that caters to various dietary preferences.

In this indulgent creation, we've carefully balanced the chocolate's allure with a mindful approach to sugar. A sugar substitute or a modest amount of natural sweeteners like honey or maple syrup elevates the cake's sweetness without overwhelming the decadence of dark chocolate.

Our Rich Dark Chocolate Beetroot Cake is perfect for showcasing the magic of chocolate and the versatility of beetroots. Whether served as an exquisite dessert or enjoyed as a luxurious afternoon treat, this cake promises a memorable experience for chocolate enthusiasts.

Ingredients:

- 1 cup almond flour or coconut flour (or a combination of both)
- 1/4 cup unsweetened cocoa powder
- 1 teaspoon baking powder
- 1/4 teaspoon salt
- 4 large eggs, at room temperature
- 1/3 cup granulated sugar substitute (e.g., stevia, erythritol) or natural sweetener (e.g., honey, maple syrup)
- 1/3 cup unsweetened applesauce or plain Greek yogurt
- 1 teaspoon pure vanilla extract
- 1 cup grated and drained raw beetroots (about 2 medium-sized beetroots)
- 1/2 cup dark chocolate chips or chopped dark chocolate

Instructions:

1. Preheat your oven to 350°F (175°C). Grease an 8-inch round cake pan and line the bottom with parchment paper.

2. In a mixing bowl, whisk together the almond flour or coconut flour (or combination), unsweetened cocoa powder, baking

powder, and salt until well combined.

3. In a separate large mixing bowl, beat the eggs and granulated sugar substitute or natural sweetener until pale and fluffy. Stir in the unsweetened applesauce or Greek yogurt and pure vanilla extract.

4. Gradually fold the dry ingredients into the egg-applesauce mixture until you have a smooth batter.

5. Gently fold in the grated and drained raw beetroots, ensuring they are evenly distributed throughout the batter.

6. Stir in the dark chocolate chips or chopped dark chocolate, adding a delightful burst of indulgence.

7. Pour the batter into the prepared cake pan and smooth the top with a spatula.

8. Bake in the preheated oven for approximately 30-35 minutes or until the cake is set and a toothpick inserted into the center comes out with moist crumbs.

9. Remove the cake from the oven and let it cool in the pan for 10 minutes. Then, carefully transfer it to a wire rack to cool completely.

10. Serve the Rich Dark Chocolate Beetroot Cake as a sumptuous dessert or as an exquisite afternoon delight.

Nutritional Information (Approximate, per serving):

- Calories: 180 kcal
- Total Fat: 14g
  - Saturated Fat: 3g
- Cholesterol: 70mg
- Sodium: 150mg
- Total Carbohydrates: 12g
  - Dietary Fiber: 3g
  - Sugars: 2g

- Protein: 7g

4.2 Black Forest Cherry Chocolate Cake

At the heart of this cake lies the richness of chocolate. Layers of moist chocolate sponge cake create the perfect canvas for the delightful medley of flavors to unfold. The intense cocoa notes intermingle with the sweetness of cherries, creating a symphony of taste that tantalizes the senses.

Cherries, with their natural sweetness and ruby-red allure, bring a burst of fruity goodness to this cake. Whether you use fresh cherries in season or opt for frozen ones, they infuse the cake with their delightful essence.

To elevate the experience of our Black Forest Cherry Chocolate Cake, we've chosen to add layers of whipped cream between the cake layers. The velvety cream adds a luxurious touch and complements the richness of chocolate and the sweetness of cherries.

For a mindful approach to sweetness, we've opted for sugar substitutes or modest amounts of natural sweeteners. This ensures that the cake remains balanced, allowing the flavors of chocolate and cherries to shine without overpowering sweetness.

Our Black Forest Cherry Chocolate Cake is perfect for special celebrations or moments when you crave an extra indulgence. It is a beautiful centerpiece that will leave your guests in awe and satisfy their desire for a luxurious and delectable dessert.

Ingredients: For the Chocolate Sponge Cake:

- 1 cup almond flour or all-purpose flour (for a gluten-containing version)

- 1/4 cup unsweetened cocoa powder

- 1 teaspoon baking powder

- 1/4 teaspoon salt

- 4 large eggs, at room temperature

- 1/3 cup granulated sugar substitute (e.g., stevia, erythritol) or natural sweetener (e.g., honey, maple syrup)

- 1/3 cup unsweetened applesauce or plain Greek yogurt

- 1 teaspoon pure vanilla extract

For the Filling and Topping:

- 1 cup pitted and halved fresh or frozen cherries

- 2 cups whipped cream (sweetened with a sugar substitute if desired)

- Dark chocolate shavings or cocoa powder, for garnish

Instructions:

For the Chocolate Sponge Cake:

1. Preheat your oven to 350°F (175°C). Grease two 8-inch round cake pans and line the bottoms with parchment paper.

2. In a mixing bowl, whisk together the almond flour or all-purpose flour, unsweetened cocoa powder, baking powder, and salt until well combined.

3. In a separate large mixing bowl, beat the eggs and granulated sugar substitute or natural sweetener until pale and fluffy. Stir in the unsweetened applesauce or Greek yogurt and pure vanilla extract.

4. Gradually fold the dry ingredients into the egg-applesauce mixture until you have a smooth batter.

5. Divide the batter evenly between the prepared cake pans and smooth the tops with a spatula.

6. Bake in the preheated oven for approximately 20-25 minutes or until the cakes are set and a toothpick inserted into the center comes out with moist crumbs.

7. Remove the cakes from the oven and let them cool in the pans for 10 minutes. Then, carefully transfer them to a wire rack to cool completely.

For the Assembly:

1. Once the cakes are completely cooled, place one cake layer on a serving plate or cake stand.

2. Spread a layer of whipped cream over the cake layer.

3. Scatter half of the halved cherries over the whipped cream.

4. Place the second cake layer on top.

5. Cover the top and sides of the cake with the remaining whipped cream.

6. Garnish the top of the cake with the remaining halved cherries and dark chocolate shavings or a dusting of cocoa powder.

7. Refrigerate the Black Forest Cherry Chocolate Cake for at least 1 hour before serving to allow the flavors to meld.

8. Slice and serve this delightful creation, and watch as your guests are captivated by the magic of Black Forest flavors.

Nutritional Information (Approximate, per serving):

- Calories: 250 kcal
- Total Fat: 18g
  - Saturated Fat: 8g
- Cholesterol: 100mg
- Sodium: 100mg
- Total Carbohydrates: 15g
  - Dietary Fiber: 2g
  - Sugars: 4g
- Protein: 7g

4.3 Hazelnut Flour Chocolate Orange Cake

Hazelnut flour, with its distinct flavor and delicate aroma, creates a delightful foundation for this cake. Its nutty essence complements the richness of chocolate, elevating the cake to a whole new level of decadence.

To enhance the delightful citrus notes, we infuse the cake with the zest of fresh oranges, adding a burst of freshness that balances the sweetness of chocolate and hazelnuts.

Our Hazelnut Flour Chocolate Orange Cake is crafted with alternative flours, making it gluten-free and suitable for those with dietary restrictions. The use of almond flour and hazelnut flour ensures a tender and moist crumb that harmonizes beautifully with the other flavors.

We've mindfully chosen sugar substitutes or natural sweeteners to maintain the cake's balance and keep the sugar content in check. This allows the flavors of chocolate and orange to shine without overwhelming sweetness.

Perfect for special occasions or as a delightful treat for afternoon tea, this cake promises to be a show-stopping centerpiece that will leave your guests in awe and delight.

Ingredients:

- 1 cup hazelnut flour
- 1 cup almond flour
- 1/4 cup unsweetened cocoa powder
- 1 teaspoon baking powder
- 1/4 teaspoon salt
- Zest of 2 oranges
- 4 large eggs, at room temperature
- 1/3 cup granulated sugar substitute (e.g., stevia, erythritol) or natural sweetener (e.g., honey, maple syrup)
- 1/3 cup unsweetened applesauce or plain Greek yogurt
- 1 teaspoon pure vanilla extract
- 1/3 cup melted dark chocolate (70% cocoa or higher)
- Optional: Orange segments and hazelnuts for garnish

Instructions:

1. Preheat your oven to 350°F (175°C). Grease an 8-inch round cake pan and line the bottom with parchment paper.

2. In a mixing bowl, whisk together the hazelnut flour, almond flour, unsweetened cocoa powder, baking powder, salt, and orange zest until well combined.

3. In a separate large mixing bowl, beat the eggs and granulated sugar substitute or natural sweetener until pale and fluffy. Stir in the unsweetened applesauce or Greek yogurt and pure vanilla extract.

4. Gradually fold the dry ingredients into the egg-applesauce mixture until you have a smooth batter.

5. Gently fold in the melted dark chocolate, ensuring it is evenly distributed throughout the batter.

6. Pour the batter into the prepared cake pan and smooth the top with a spatula.

7. Bake in the preheated oven for approximately 25-30 minutes or until the cake is set and a toothpick inserted into the center comes out with moist crumbs.

8. Remove the cake from the oven and let it cool in the pan for 10 minutes. Then, carefully transfer it to a wire rack to cool completely.

9. Once the cake is completely cooled, garnish with orange segments and hazelnuts for an elegant finish.

10. Serve the Hazelnut Flour Chocolate Orange Cake as a delightful dessert or a sumptuous addition to afternoon tea.

Nutritional Information (Approximate, per serving):

- Calories: 220 kcal
- Total Fat: 16g
  - Saturated Fat: 4g
- Cholesterol: 70mg

- Sodium: 100mg
- Total Carbohydrates: 14g
  - Dietary Fiber: 3g
  - Sugars: 2g
- Protein: 7g

UNIQUE SPECIAL OCCASION CAKES

These cakes are crafted to be the centerpiece of your most cherished celebrations. Whether you're commemorating a milestone birthday, a joyous wedding, a heartwarming anniversary, or any other special occasion, these unique creations will add a touch of magic to your festivities.

Each cake in this chapter is a masterpiece of artistry and flavor, designed to leave a lasting impression on your guests and create unforgettable memories. From stunning tiered cakes adorned with intricate decorations to whimsical designs that reflect your personality, these creations are a testament to the boundless possibilities of baking.

Our unique special occasion cakes encompass a delightful variety of flavors, textures, and ingredients. Explore the richness of fruit-based cakes, the indulgence of chocolate delights, and the elegance of floral-inspired creations. From flourless wonders to low-sugar marvels, these cakes embrace a mindful approach to baking without compromising on taste or splendor.

Every cake is an expression of creativity, skill, and love, carefully crafted to celebrate life's most precious moments. Embrace the joy of baking as you embark on a journey through the realm of unique special occasion cakes, where each slice is a celebration of love, happiness, and togetherness.

5.1 Sugar-Free Red Velvet Cake

The vibrant red hue of the cake, achieved by a delicate balance of cocoa powder and food coloring, is an instant visual delight. But what truly sets this cake apart is its delectable taste and texture.

The cake's moist and velvety crumb, achieved through the careful blending of alternative flours, ensures a delightful eating experience. Almond flour and coconut flour work together to create a gluten-free masterpiece that caters to various dietary preferences.

In place of refined sugar, we utilize sugar substitutes or natural sweeteners to enhance the cake's sweetness. This thoughtful approach allows you to enjoy the classic red velvet flavors without the impact on blood sugar levels.

To maintain the cake's characteristic richness, we top it with a luscious cream cheese frosting that strikes the perfect balance between tangy and sweet. The frosting complements the cake's flavors, creating a heavenly duo that is hard to resist.

Our Sugar-Free Red Velvet Cake is perfect for celebrating special occasions or simply savoring a guilt-free treat. Whether you're sharing it with friends, family, or enjoying a quiet moment of indulgence, this cake promises to delight your senses and leave you wanting more.

Ingredients: For the Red Velvet Cake:

- 1 cup almond flour

- 1/4 cup coconut flour

- 1/4 cup unsweetened cocoa powder

- 1 teaspoon baking powder

- 1/4 teaspoon baking soda

- 1/4 teaspoon salt

- 4 large eggs, at room temperature

- 1/3 cup granulated sugar substitute (e.g., stevia, erythritol) or natural sweetener (e.g., honey, maple syrup)

- 1/3 cup unsweetened applesauce or plain Greek yogurt

- 1/4 cup unsweetened almond milk or any milk of your choice

- 1 teaspoon pure vanilla extract

- Red food coloring (gel or liquid), as needed

For the Cream Cheese Frosting:

- 8 ounces cream cheese, softened

- 1/4 cup unsalted butter, softened

- 1/3 cup powdered sugar substitute (e.g., powdered erythritol)

- 1 teaspoon pure vanilla extract

Instructions:

For the Red Velvet Cake:

1. Preheat your oven to 350°F (175°C). Grease two 8-inch round cake pans and line the bottoms with parchment paper.

2. In a mixing bowl, whisk together the almond flour, coconut flour, unsweetened cocoa powder, baking powder, baking soda, and salt until well combined.

3. In a separate large mixing bowl, beat the eggs and granulated sugar substitute or natural sweetener until pale and fluffy. Stir in the unsweetened applesauce or Greek yogurt, unsweetened almond milk, and pure vanilla extract.

4. Gradually fold the dry ingredients into the egg mixture until you have a smooth batter.

5. Add red food coloring as needed to achieve the desired vibrant red hue. Start with a small amount and adjust to your preference.

6. Divide the batter evenly between the prepared cake pans and smooth the tops with a spatula.

7. Bake in the preheated oven for approximately 25-30 minutes or until the cakes are set and a toothpick inserted into the center comes out with moist crumbs.

8. Remove the cakes from the oven and let them cool in the pans for 10 minutes. Then, carefully transfer them to a wire rack to cool completely.

For the Cream Cheese Frosting:

1. In a mixing bowl, beat the softened cream cheese and unsalted butter until smooth and creamy.

2. Gradually add the powdered sugar substitute and pure vanilla extract. Continue to beat until the frosting is well combined and fluffy.

Assembly:

1. Once the cakes are completely cooled, place one cake layer on a serving plate or cake stand.

2. Spread a layer of cream cheese frosting over the cake layer.

3. Place the second cake layer on top.

4. Cover the top and sides of the cake with the remaining cream cheese frosting.

5. If desired, use a spatula or cake scraper to create decorative swirls or patterns on the frosting.

6. Refrigerate the Sugar-Free Red Velvet Cake for at least 1 hour before serving to allow the flavors to meld.

7. Slice and serve this delightful creation, and enjoy the classic allure of red velvet without the guilt of added sugar.

Nutritional Information (Approximate, per serving):

- Calories: 180 kcal
- Total Fat: 14g
  - Saturated Fat: 7g
- Cholesterol: 90mg
- Sodium: 150mg
- Total Carbohydrates: 10g
  - Dietary Fiber: 2g

- Sugars: 1g

- Protein: 5g

5.2 Pistachio Rosewater Celebration Cake

At the heart of this cake lies the rich and nutty flavor of pistachios, finely ground to create a tender and moist crumb. The subtle earthiness of pistachios is beautifully complemented by the delicate fragrance of rosewater, infusing each bite with a touch of floral wonder.

The beauty of this cake extends to its presentation, adorned with a luscious rosewater buttercream frosting that carries the essence of roses and elevates the cake's elegance. The frosting's velvety texture is a perfect match for the tender crumb, creating a harmonious blend of flavors and mouthfeel.

To make this cake even more special, we've added a touch of edible rose petals as a delightful garnish, adding a visual allure that will captivate your guests.

Our Pistachio Rosewater Celebration Cake is a work of art that complements any joyous occasion. Whether you're celebrating a wedding, an anniversary, or any other momentous event, this cake promises to be the highlight of the celebration, creating an unforgettable experience for you and your guests.

Ingredients: For the Pistachio Cake:

- 1 cup shelled pistachios, unsalted

- 1 cup almond flour

- 1/4 cup all-purpose flour (or gluten-free flour blend)

- 1 teaspoon baking powder

- 1/4 teaspoon salt

- 4 large eggs, at room temperature

- 1/2 cup granulated sugar substitute (e.g., stevia, erythritol) or natural sweetener (e.g., honey, maple syrup)

- 1/2 cup unsweetened applesauce or plain Greek yogurt

- 1 teaspoon pure vanilla extract
- 1/2 teaspoon rosewater

For the Rosewater Buttercream Frosting:

- 1 cup unsalted butter, softened
- 3 cups powdered sugar substitute (e.g., powdered erythritol)
- 1 teaspoon pure vanilla extract
- 1/2 teaspoon rosewater
- Pink or rose food coloring (gel or liquid), as needed
- Edible rose petals, for garnish (optional)

Instructions:

For the Pistachio Cake:

1. Preheat your oven to 350°F (175°C). Grease two 8-inch round cake pans and line the bottoms with parchment paper.

2. In a food processor, pulse the shelled pistachios until finely ground, resembling a coarse flour.

3. In a mixing bowl, whisk together the ground pistachios, almond flour, all-purpose flour (or gluten-free flour blend), baking powder, and salt until well combined.

4. In a separate large mixing bowl, beat the eggs and granulated sugar substitute or natural sweetener until pale and fluffy. Stir in the unsweetened applesauce or Greek yogurt, pure vanilla extract, and rosewater.

5. Gradually fold the dry ingredients into the egg mixture until you have a smooth batter.

6. Divide the batter evenly between the prepared cake pans and smooth the tops with a spatula.

7. Bake in the preheated oven for approximately 25-30 minutes or until the cakes are set and a toothpick inserted into the center comes out with moist crumbs.

8. Remove the cakes from the oven and let them cool in the pans

for 10 minutes. Then, carefully transfer them to a wire rack to cool completely.

For the Rosewater Buttercream Frosting:

1. In a mixing bowl, beat the softened butter until smooth and creamy.

2. Gradually add the powdered sugar substitute, pure vanilla extract, and rosewater. Continue to beat until the frosting is well combined and fluffy.

3. Add pink or rose food coloring as needed to achieve the desired pastel hue. Start with a small amount and adjust to your preference.

Assembly:

1. Once the cakes are completely cooled, place one cake layer on a serving plate or cake stand.

2. Spread a layer of rosewater buttercream frosting over the cake layer.

3. Place the second cake layer on top.

4. Cover the top and sides of the cake with the remaining rosewater buttercream frosting.

5. If desired, use a spatula or cake scraper to create decorative swirls or patterns on the frosting.

6. Garnish the cake with edible rose petals for an exquisite finish.

7. Refrigerate the Pistachio Rosewater Celebration Cake for at least 1 hour before serving to allow the flavors to meld.

8. Slice and serve this enchanting creation, and let the captivating flavors and beauty of roses transport you to a realm of celebration and wonder.

Nutritional Information (Approximate, per serving):

- Calories: 320 kcal

- Total Fat: 24g

- Saturated Fat: 12g

- Cholesterol: 110mg

- Sodium: 150mg

- Total Carbohydrates: 24g

  - Dietary Fiber: 3g

  - Sugars: 1g

- Protein: 6g

5.3 Guilt-Free Coffee and Walnut Cake

The star of this cake is the bold and aromatic coffee, infusing each bite with a comforting warmth that coffee enthusiasts will adore. Whether you prefer the intensity of espresso or the smoothness of brewed coffee, this cake embraces the versatility of coffee flavors.

To enhance the nutritional profile and add a delightful crunch, we've incorporated chopped walnuts throughout the cake. Walnuts not only complement the coffee flavors but also offer a wealth of health benefits, making this cake a nutritious option for your dessert table.

Our Guilt-Free Coffee and Walnut Cake is thoughtfully crafted with alternative flours, such as almond flour or coconut flour, to make it gluten-free and suitable for various dietary needs.

To maintain a mindful approach to sweetness, we've chosen sugar substitutes or natural sweeteners, ensuring that you can savor the cake's flavors without added guilt.

Perfect for a midday treat, an afternoon pick-me-up, or a delightful dessert, this cake will bring joy to your coffee breaks and special occasions alike.

Ingredients:

- 1 cup almond flour or coconut flour (or a combination of both)

- 1/4 cup unsweetened cocoa powder

- 1 teaspoon baking powder

- 1/4 teaspoon salt

- 4 large eggs, at room temperature

- 1/3 cup granulated sugar substitute (e.g., stevia, erythritol) or natural sweetener (e.g., honey, maple syrup)

- 1/3 cup unsweetened applesauce or plain Greek yogurt

- 1/4 cup strong brewed coffee or espresso, cooled

- 1 teaspoon pure vanilla extract

- 1/2 cup chopped walnuts

Instructions:

1. Preheat your oven to 350°F (175°C). Grease an 8-inch round cake pan and line the bottom with parchment paper.

2. In a mixing bowl, whisk together the almond flour or coconut flour (or combination), unsweetened cocoa powder, baking powder, and salt until well combined.

3. In a separate large mixing bowl, beat the eggs and granulated sugar substitute or natural sweetener until pale and fluffy. Stir in the unsweetened applesauce or Greek yogurt, brewed coffee or espresso, and pure vanilla extract.

4. Gradually fold the dry ingredients into the egg-coffee mixture until you have a smooth batter.

5. Gently fold in the chopped walnuts, ensuring they are evenly distributed throughout the batter.

6. Pour the batter into the prepared cake pan and smooth the top with a spatula.

7. Bake in the preheated oven for approximately 25-30 minutes or until the cake is set and a toothpick inserted into the center comes out with moist crumbs.

8. Remove the cake from the oven and let it cool in the pan for 10 minutes. Then, carefully transfer it to a wire rack to cool completely.

9. Serve the Guilt-Free Coffee and Walnut Cake as a delightful

treat for coffee lovers or as a guilt-free dessert for any occasion.

Nutritional Information (Approximate, per serving):

- Calories: 200 kcal
- Total Fat: 16g
    - Saturated Fat: 4g
- Cholesterol: 70mg
- Sodium: 150mg
- Total Carbohydrates: 10g
    - Dietary Fiber: 3g
    - Sugars: 1g
- Protein: 8g

DECADENT CHEESECAKES

Cheesecakes are a timeless classic that have stood the test of time, winning the affections of dessert enthusiasts for generations. With their velvety-smooth texture, rich flavors, and endless possibilities for creativity, cheesecakes hold a special place in the hearts of dessert lovers everywhere.

Each cheesecake in this chapter is a celebration of decadence, meticulously crafted to showcase a range of indulgent flavors and innovative combinations. From traditional New York-style cheesecakes to exotic variations inspired by world cuisines, this collection offers a delightful array of choices to suit every palate.

Every recipe is designed to be a show-stopping centerpiece for your celebrations or simply a luxurious treat for moments of self-indulgence. From the first luscious bite to the last, these cheesecakes promise to transport you to a world of pure delight, where the pleasures of creamy goodness abound.

Discover the magic of creamy textures, exquisite flavors, and tantalizing toppings that make these cheesecakes an experience to cherish. Whether you're a seasoned baker or a dessert enthusiast looking to explore the art of cheesecake-making, this chapter holds the keys to creating unforgettable culinary delights.

6.1 Low-Carb Raspberry Swirl Cheesecake

At the heart of this cheesecake lies the velvety-smooth cream cheese filling, exquisitely balanced to achieve a creamy texture that melts in your mouth. We've carefully chosen sugar substitutes or natural sweeteners to add just the right amount of sweetness, without compromising on the dessert's delectable charm.

To infuse the cake with vibrant raspberry flavor, we create a swirl of raspberry puree that not only adds a beautiful visual appeal but also imparts a burst of fruity goodness with every bite.

Our Low-Carb Raspberry Swirl Cheesecake is thoughtfully designed to be gluten-free, making it a delightful option for those with dietary restrictions or those looking to reduce gluten in their diets.

This cheesecake is perfect for special occasions or whenever you crave an indulgent treat with a mindful twist. Each slice promises to transport you to a world of creamy bliss and fruity delight, as you embrace the magic of a low-carb dessert that doesn't compromise on taste.

Ingredients: For the Crust:

- 1 1/2 cups almond flour
- 1/4 cup unsweetened cocoa powder
- 1/4 cup granulated sugar substitute (e.g., stevia, erythritol) or natural sweetener (e.g., honey, maple syrup)
- 1/3 cup unsalted butter, melted

For the Cheesecake Filling:

- 24 ounces cream cheese, softened
- 1/2 cup granulated sugar substitute (e.g., stevia, erythritol) or natural sweetener (e.g., honey, maple syrup)
- 3 large eggs, at room temperature
- 1 teaspoon pure vanilla extract
- 1/3 cup plain Greek yogurt or sour cream

- 1/2 cup raspberry puree (made from fresh or frozen raspberries)

Instructions:

For the Crust:

1. Preheat your oven to 350°F (175°C). Grease a 9-inch springform pan and line the bottom with parchment paper.

2. In a mixing bowl, combine the almond flour, unsweetened cocoa powder, and granulated sugar substitute or natural sweetener.

3. Stir in the melted butter until the mixture resembles wet sand.

4. Press the crust mixture evenly into the bottom of the prepared springform pan, creating a firm and compact crust.

5. Bake the crust in the preheated oven for 8-10 minutes, or until it is set and slightly firm to the touch. Remove from the oven and let it cool while preparing the filling.

For the Cheesecake Filling:

1. In a large mixing bowl, beat the softened cream cheese and granulated sugar substitute or natural sweetener until smooth and creamy.

2. Add the eggs one at a time, beating well after each addition.

3. Stir in the pure vanilla extract and plain Greek yogurt or sour cream until fully incorporated.

4. Pour the cheesecake filling over the cooled crust in the springform pan.

5. Drop spoonfuls of raspberry puree onto the cheesecake filling. Use a knife or skewer to gently swirl the raspberry puree into the filling to create a marbled effect.

6. Place the springform pan on a baking sheet (to catch any potential leaks) and bake the cheesecake in the preheated oven for approximately 40-45 minutes or until the edges are set and the center is slightly jiggly.

7. Turn off the oven, crack the oven door open, and let the

cheesecake cool in the oven for an additional 1-2 hours.

8. Once the cheesecake has cooled, refrigerate it for at least 4 hours or overnight to set.

9. Before serving, carefully remove the sides of the springform pan.

10. Slice and serve this delightful Low-Carb Raspberry Swirl Cheesecake, and enjoy the blissful combination of creamy richness and tangy raspberry flavor in every bite.

Nutritional Information (Approximate, per serving):

- Calories: 350 kcal

- Total Fat: 30g

    - Saturated Fat: 14g

- Cholesterol: 130mg

- Sodium: 220mg

- Total Carbohydrates: 10g

    - Dietary Fiber: 3g

    - Sugars: 2g

- Protein: 10g

6.2 Lemon and Ginger Greek Yogurt Cheesecake

Experience a burst of zesty freshness and a hint of spiciness with our Lemon and Ginger Greek Yogurt Cheesecake—a delightful fusion of flavors that will awaken your senses and leave you craving more. This cheesecake is a celebration of citrusy tanginess, balanced with the warm, earthy notes of ginger, and elevated with the lusciousness of Greek yogurt.

The star of this cheesecake is the velvety Greek yogurt, which not only adds creaminess but also provides a tangy twist to the classic cheesecake. Greek yogurt is known for its probiotic benefits and nutritional value, making this dessert a healthier option without compromising on flavor.

To add depth to the flavor profile, we infuse the cheesecake with the bright essence of fresh lemon zest and juice. The zingy lemon notes complement the tangy yogurt, creating a harmonious medley that is both refreshing and indulgent.

The addition of ground ginger adds a touch of warmth and a pleasant spiciness, elevating the flavors to a new level of complexity. The result is a cheesecake that is both soothing and invigorating, making it a perfect choice for any occasion.

Our Lemon and Ginger Greek Yogurt Cheesecake is designed to be lighter and less sweet, making it ideal for those who appreciate a more subtle sweetness or are conscious of their sugar intake.

Ingredients: For the Crust:

- 1 1/2 cups almond flour

- 1/4 cup unsalted butter, melted

- 1/4 cup granulated sugar substitute (e.g., stevia, erythritol) or natural sweetener (e.g., honey, maple syrup)

- 1 teaspoon ground ginger

For the Cheesecake Filling:

- 24 ounces cream cheese, softened

- 1 cup plain Greek yogurt

- 1/2 cup granulated sugar substitute (e.g., stevia, erythritol) or natural sweetener (e.g., honey, maple syrup)

- 3 large eggs, at room temperature

- Zest of 1 large lemon

- 1/4 cup fresh lemon juice

- 1 teaspoon pure vanilla extract

- 1 teaspoon ground ginger

Instructions:

For the Crust:

1. Preheat your oven to 350°F (175°C). Grease a 9-inch

springform pan and line the bottom with parchment paper.

2. In a mixing bowl, combine the almond flour, melted butter, granulated sugar substitute or natural sweetener, and ground ginger. Mix until the ingredients are well combined and the mixture resembles wet sand.

3. Press the crust mixture evenly into the bottom of the prepared springform pan, creating a firm and compact crust.

4. Bake the crust in the preheated oven for 10 minutes or until it is set and slightly golden. Remove from the oven and let it cool while preparing the filling.

For the Cheesecake Filling:

1. In a large mixing bowl, beat the softened cream cheese and granulated sugar substitute or natural sweetener until smooth and creamy.

2. Add the Greek yogurt, and continue to beat until fully incorporated and the mixture is smooth.

3. Beat in the eggs, one at a time, until fully combined.

4. Stir in the lemon zest, fresh lemon juice, pure vanilla extract, and ground ginger until well incorporated.

5. Pour the cheesecake filling over the cooled crust in the springform pan.

6. Smooth the top with a spatula for an even surface.

7. Bake the cheesecake in the preheated oven for approximately 40-45 minutes or until the edges are set, and the center is slightly jiggly.

8. Turn off the oven, crack the oven door open, and let the cheesecake cool in the oven for an additional 1-2 hours.

9. Once the cheesecake has cooled, refrigerate it for at least 4 hours or overnight to set.

10. Before serving, carefully remove the sides of the springform pan.

11. Slice and serve this delightful Lemon and Ginger Greek Yogurt

Cheesecake, and enjoy the invigorating combination of lemon and ginger paired with the velvety creaminess of Greek yogurt in every blissful bite.

Nutritional Information (Approximate, per serving):

- Calories: 320 kcal
- Total Fat: 28g
  - Saturated Fat: 13g
- Cholesterol: 120mg
- Sodium: 200mg
- Total Carbohydrates: 8g
  - Dietary Fiber: 2g
  - Sugars: 2g
- Protein: 10g

6.3 White Chocolate and Raspberry Cheesecake

At the heart of this cheesecake is the luscious white chocolate, delicately melted into the cream cheese filling to create a smooth and creamy texture that is simply divine. The white chocolate adds a touch of elegance and elevates the dessert to a whole new level of sophistication.

To complement the sweetness of white chocolate, we infuse the cheesecake with a delightful swirl of raspberry puree, creating a visually stunning effect and imparting a refreshing tanginess to each delectable bite.

The combination of sweet and tart, smooth and creamy, makes this cheesecake a perfect choice for special occasions or any time you crave a truly indulgent treat. Each slice promises to transport you to a world of blissful pleasure, where the magic of white chocolate and the allure of raspberries create a symphony of flavors that will leave you utterly enchanted.

Our White Chocolate and Raspberry Cheesecake is crafted with the finest ingredients, making it an exquisite dessert that deserves a place at the center of your dessert table.

Ingredients: For the Crust:

- 1 1/2 cups graham cracker crumbs (or almond flour for a gluten-free version)
- 1/4 cup granulated sugar substitute (e.g., stevia, erythritol) or natural sweetener (e.g., honey, maple syrup)
- 1/3 cup unsalted butter, melted

For the Cheesecake Filling:

- 24 ounces cream cheese, softened
- 1 cup white chocolate chips, melted and cooled
- 1/2 cup granulated sugar substitute (e.g., stevia, erythritol) or natural sweetener (e.g., honey, maple syrup)
- 3 large eggs, at room temperature
- 1 teaspoon pure vanilla extract
- 1/2 cup raspberry puree (made from fresh or frozen raspberries)

Instructions:

For the Crust:

1. Preheat your oven to 350°F (175°C). Grease a 9-inch springform pan and line the bottom with parchment paper.

2. In a mixing bowl, combine the graham cracker crumbs (or almond flour), granulated sugar substitute or natural sweetener, and melted butter. Mix until the ingredients are well combined and the mixture resembles wet sand.

3. Press the crust mixture evenly into the bottom of the prepared springform pan, creating a firm and compact crust.

4. Bake the crust in the preheated oven for 8-10 minutes or until it is set and lightly golden. Remove from the oven and let it cool while preparing the filling.

For the Cheesecake Filling:

1. In a double boiler or microwave, melt the white chocolate chips until smooth. Let the melted white chocolate cool slightly.

2. In a large mixing bowl, beat the softened cream cheese and granulated sugar substitute or natural sweetener until smooth and creamy.

3. Stir in the melted white chocolate until fully incorporated and the mixture is smooth.

4. Beat in the eggs, one at a time, until fully combined.

5. Stir in the pure vanilla extract until well incorporated.

6. Pour the cheesecake filling over the cooled crust in the springform pan.

7. Drop spoonfuls of raspberry puree onto the cheesecake filling. Use a knife or skewer to gently swirl the raspberry puree into the filling to create a marbled effect.

8. Place the springform pan on a baking sheet (to catch any potential leaks) and bake the cheesecake in the preheated oven for approximately 40-45 minutes or until the edges are set, and the center is slightly jiggly.

9. Turn off the oven, crack the oven door open, and let the cheesecake cool in the oven for an additional 1-2 hours.

10. Once the cheesecake has cooled, refrigerate it for at least 4 hours or overnight to set.

11. Before serving, carefully remove the sides of the springform pan.

12. Slice and serve this luxurious White Chocolate and Raspberry Cheesecake, and delight in the divine combination of white chocolate and raspberries in every heavenly bite.

Nutritional Information (Approximate, per serving):

- Calories: 380 kcal

- Total Fat: 30g

- Saturated Fat: 16g
- Cholesterol: 120mg
- Sodium: 240mg
- Total Carbohydrates: 20g
  - Dietary Fiber: 2g
  - Sugars: 10g
- Protein: 8g

SAVORY AND SAVORY-SWEET CAKES

Cakes have long been associated with sweet indulgence, but this chapter celebrates the versatility of cakes as a canvas for savory delights. From the subtle charm of herb-infused cakes to the unexpected allure of savory-sweet combinations, we showcase a range of recipes that cater to adventurous taste buds and culinary enthusiasts alike.

Each savory and savory-sweet cake in this collection is thoughtfully crafted to offer a delightful alternative to traditional sweet treats. Savory cakes encompass a variety of ingredients, including cheeses, vegetables, meats, and a medley of herbs and spices, creating a harmonious blend of flavors that awaken the senses and challenge the norm.

Incorporating these savory delights into your culinary repertoire opens a world of possibilities for breakfasts, brunches, light lunches, or as an accompaniment to soups and salads. These cakes offer a new dimension to your dining experiences, making any meal an occasion for culinary exploration.

Our savory and savory-sweet cakes are a delightful addition to your repertoire, ensuring that you can surprise and impress your guests with flavors they may have never imagined in a cake. Let your creativity flourish as you experiment with savory ingredients, elevating your baking to new heights of sophistication and innovation.

7.1 Savory Mediterranean Olive and Herb Cake

At the heart of this cake is a harmonious blend of Kalamata olives, known for their rich and distinctive flavor, and a medley of fragrant herbs like rosemary, thyme, and oregano. These savory elements infuse the cake with a depth of flavor that is both comforting and invigorating.

The moist and tender crumb of the cake is achieved through a carefully balanced combination of olive oil and Greek yogurt, adding a touch of creaminess that complements the savory profile.

Our Savory Mediterranean Olive and Herb Cake is a delightful option for brunch, picnics, or as an accompaniment to a Mediterranean-inspired meal. Serve it as an appetizer, slice it for a light lunch, or savor it alongside a fresh Greek salad to immerse yourself in the full Mediterranean experience.

The cake is versatile and open to your creative flair—experiment with different olives, herbs, or even add crumbled feta cheese for an extra burst of Mediterranean delight.

Ingredients:

- 1 1/2 cups all-purpose flour
- 1 1/2 teaspoons baking powder
- 1/2 teaspoon baking soda
- 1/2 teaspoon salt
- 1/4 cup extra-virgin olive oil
- 1 cup Greek yogurt
- 3 large eggs, at room temperature
- 1 cup pitted Kalamata olives, chopped
- 1 tablespoon fresh rosemary, finely chopped
- 1 tablespoon fresh thyme leaves
- 1 tablespoon fresh oregano, finely chopped

- Zest of 1 lemon

Instructions:

1. Preheat your oven to 350°F (175°C). Grease a 9x5-inch loaf pan and line the bottom with parchment paper.

2. In a medium mixing bowl, whisk together the all-purpose flour, baking powder, baking soda, and salt until well combined.

3. In a separate large mixing bowl, whisk together the olive oil, Greek yogurt, and eggs until smooth.

4. Gradually add the dry ingredients to the wet ingredients and mix until just combined.

5. Gently fold in the chopped Kalamata olives, fresh rosemary, thyme leaves, oregano, and lemon zest.

6. Pour the batter into the prepared loaf pan and smooth the top with a spatula.

7. Bake in the preheated oven for approximately 40-45 minutes or until a toothpick inserted into the center comes out clean.

8. Remove the cake from the oven and let it cool in the pan for 10 minutes. Then, transfer it to a wire rack to cool completely.

9. Slice the Savory Mediterranean Olive and Herb Cake and serve it with a drizzle of extra-virgin olive oil or a dollop of Greek yogurt. Enjoy this delightful creation as an appetizer, a light lunch, or a Mediterranean-inspired accompaniment to your meal.

Nutritional Information (Approximate, per serving):

- Calories: 220 kcal
- Total Fat: 12g
  - Saturated Fat: 2g
- Cholesterol: 60mg
- Sodium: 400mg
- Total Carbohydrates: 22g

- Dietary Fiber: 1g
- Sugars: 1g
- Protein: 6g

7.2 Cornbread with Cheddar and Jalapenos

At the core of this cornbread is the golden goodness of cornmeal, which infuses the cake with a subtly sweet and nutty flavor, evoking memories of warm Southern kitchens and homestyle cooking.

We elevate the cornbread to new heights with the addition of sharp cheddar cheese, which melts beautifully into the crumb, adding a delightful creaminess and a tangy undertone that perfectly balances the jalapenos' spiciness.

Speaking of jalapenos, their vibrant and peppery essence adds a pleasant heat to the cornbread, enhancing the overall flavor profile and giving it a Tex-Mex twist that is both comforting and exciting.

Our Cornbread with Cheddar and Jalapenos is a versatile addition to your culinary repertoire. Serve it as a side dish to complement your favorite Tex-Mex meals, or enjoy it on its own as a delectable snack. The texture is moist yet slightly crumbly, making it a delightful companion to soups, stews, and chili.

Ingredients:

- 1 cup yellow cornmeal
- 1 cup all-purpose flour
- 1/4 cup granulated sugar
- 1 tablespoon baking powder
- 1 teaspoon salt
- 1 cup buttermilk
- 1/4 cup unsalted butter, melted and cooled
- 2 large eggs, at room temperature
- 1 cup sharp cheddar cheese, shredded

- 2 jalapeno peppers, seeded and finely chopped

Instructions:

1. Preheat your oven to 375°F (190°C). Grease an 8x8-inch baking pan or a 9-inch cast-iron skillet.

2. In a large mixing bowl, whisk together the cornmeal, all-purpose flour, granulated sugar, baking powder, and salt until well combined.

3. In a separate mixing bowl, whisk together the buttermilk, melted butter, and eggs until smooth.

4. Gradually add the wet ingredients to the dry ingredients, and mix until just combined.

5. Gently fold in the shredded cheddar cheese and chopped jalapenos until evenly distributed throughout the batter.

6. Pour the batter into the prepared baking pan or skillet and smooth the top with a spatula.

7. Bake in the preheated oven for approximately 25-30 minutes or until a toothpick inserted into the center comes out clean.

8. Remove the cornbread from the oven and let it cool in the pan for 10 minutes. Then, transfer it to a wire rack to cool completely.

9. Slice the Cornbread with Cheddar and Jalapenos and serve it warm or at room temperature. Enjoy this savory delight as a side dish or a delightful snack that brings the flavors of Tex-Mex cuisine to your table.

Nutritional Information (Approximate, per serving):

- Calories: 210 kcal
- Total Fat: 9g
  - Saturated Fat: 5g
- Cholesterol: 60mg
- Sodium: 380mg
- Total Carbohydrates: 25g

- Dietary Fiber: 1g

- Sugars: 6g

- Protein: 7g

7.3 Sweet Potato and Pecan Cake

Experience the cozy charm of autumn in every bite with our Sweet Potato and Pecan Cake—a delightful creation that celebrates the rich flavors of sweet potatoes and the nutty goodness of pecans. This savory-sweet cake is a celebration of seasonal delights, where the earthy sweetness of roasted sweet potatoes meets the buttery crunch of toasted pecans, creating a taste experience that is both comforting and indulgent.

At the heart of this cake lies the sweet potato, roasted to perfection to intensify its natural sweetness and enhance its velvety texture. The sweet potato imparts a delightful moistness to the cake, making each slice a decadent treat that will warm your heart and soul.

To elevate the flavors, we generously sprinkle the cake with toasted pecans, adding a satisfying crunch and a warm nuttiness that complements the sweet potatoes beautifully.

The subtle sweetness of the cake is enhanced by a medley of warm spices like cinnamon and nutmeg, creating a symphony of flavors that evoke memories of cozy gatherings and cherished moments.

Our Sweet Potato and Pecan Cake is the epitome of autumnal indulgence. Serve it as a dessert for special occasions or enjoy it with a cup of hot tea or coffee as a delightful afternoon treat.

Ingredients:

- 1 cup all-purpose flour

- 1 teaspoon baking powder

- 1/2 teaspoon baking soda

- 1/2 teaspoon salt

- 1 teaspoon ground cinnamon

- 1/4 teaspoon ground nutmeg
- 1 cup roasted and mashed sweet potatoes (about 2 medium sweet potatoes)
- 1/2 cup unsalted butter, melted and cooled
- 1/2 cup granulated sugar
- 1/2 cup packed brown sugar
- 2 large eggs, at room temperature
- 1 teaspoon pure vanilla extract
- 1/2 cup buttermilk
- 1/2 cup chopped pecans, toasted

Instructions:

1. Preheat your oven to 350°F (175°C). Grease and flour a 9-inch round cake pan or line it with parchment paper.

2. In a medium mixing bowl, whisk together the all-purpose flour, baking powder, baking soda, salt, ground cinnamon, and ground nutmeg until well combined.

3. In a separate large mixing bowl, whisk together the roasted and mashed sweet potatoes, melted butter, granulated sugar, and brown sugar until smooth.

4. Beat in the eggs, one at a time, until fully combined.

5. Stir in the pure vanilla extract.

6. Gradually add the dry ingredients to the wet ingredients, alternating with the buttermilk, and mix until just combined.

7. Gently fold in the chopped pecans until evenly distributed throughout the batter.

8. Pour the batter into the prepared cake pan and smooth the top with a spatula.

9. Bake in the preheated oven for approximately 30-35 minutes or until a toothpick inserted into the center comes out clean.

10. Remove the cake from the oven and let it cool in the pan for 10

minutes. Then, transfer it to a wire rack to cool completely.

11. Slice the Sweet Potato and Pecan Cake and serve it warm or at room temperature. Enjoy this delightful creation as a dessert for special occasions or a cozy treat to embrace the flavors of autumn.

Nutritional Information (Approximate, per serving):

- Calories: 270 kcal
- Total Fat: 14g
  - Saturated Fat: 7g
- Cholesterol: 60mg
- Sodium: 220mg
- Total Carbohydrates: 33g
  - Dietary Fiber: 2g
  - Sugars: 19g
- Protein: 3g

FROSTINGS AND GLAZES

Frostings and glazes are the crowning jewels that transform ordinary cakes into extraordinary creations. Each recipe is thoughtfully crafted to complement a variety of cake flavors, from classic vanilla and chocolate to fruity delights and nutty treats.

From the smooth and silky textures of buttercream to the glossy and vibrant allure of fruit glazes, these creations allow you to express your artistic flair and enhance the flavors of your favorite cakes.

Whether you seek a showstopping dessert for a special occasion or a simple pleasure to elevate everyday moments, this chapter offers an array of choices that cater to your preferences and creative vision.

Each frosting and glaze brings a unique character to the table, creating a delightful symphony of flavors that harmonize with the essence of the cake.

9.1 Sugar-Free Cream Cheese Frosting

At the heart of this frosting lies the velvety smoothness of cream cheese, which provides a delightful tanginess and a luxurious mouthfeel that elevates any cake to new heights.

To achieve the perfect level of sweetness, we employ natural sweeteners such as stevia or erythritol, ensuring that every spoonful delivers a delicious sweetness without the need for refined sugars.

The result is a luscious and creamy frosting that pairs exceptionally well with a variety of cakes, from classic carrot cake to red velvet and everything in between.

Our Sugar-Free Cream Cheese Frosting is the epitome of a health-conscious indulgence, offering a guilt-free option for those seeking a sugar-free lifestyle or managing diabetes without sacrificing the joys of frosting.

Serve this frosting atop your favorite cakes or use it as a delicious dip for fruit platters. The possibilities are endless, and every bite will leave you craving more of this delectable creation.

Ingredients:

- 8 oz (225g) cream cheese, softened
- 1/2 cup unsalted butter, softened
- 1 teaspoon pure vanilla extract
- 1/4 teaspoon salt
- 1/2 teaspoon liquid stevia or erythritol (adjust to taste)
- 1-2 tablespoons milk or plant-based milk (as needed for consistency)

Instructions:

1. In a mixing bowl, beat the softened cream cheese and unsalted butter until smooth and well combined.

2. Add the pure vanilla extract and salt to the bowl, and continue to beat until incorporated.

3. Gradually add the liquid stevia or erythritol, adjusting the amount to achieve your desired level of sweetness. Remember to taste as you go to ensure it matches your preference.

4. If the frosting is too thick, add a tablespoon of milk or plant-based milk at a time, and continue beating until the desired consistency is reached.

5. Once the Sugar-Free Cream Cheese Frosting reaches your desired texture and sweetness, it is ready to use.

6. Spread the frosting generously over your favorite cake, or use it as a delectable dip for fruit platters.

Note: You can adjust the sweetness and texture of the frosting based on your personal preferences. If you prefer a stiffer frosting for piping, use less milk or plant-based milk. For a smoother and creamier texture, add more liquid.

9.2 Vegan Chocolate Ganache

At the core of this ganache lies the magic of dairy-free chocolate, chosen for its smooth texture and rich cocoa flavor. Combined with the lusciousness of coconut milk, this ganache achieves a silky and glossy consistency that is ideal for glazing cakes, filling cupcakes, or simply drizzling over your favorite desserts.

The best part of this Vegan Chocolate Ganache is that it requires minimal effort and ingredients, yet delivers maximum flavor and elegance.

Our Vegan Chocolate Ganache is the epitome of indulgence without compromise, offering a delectable option for those following a vegan lifestyle or seeking a dairy-free alternative to classic ganache.

Serve this ganache as a luscious glaze for cakes, a dip for fruits, or a drizzle for cookies and pastries. Each spoonful will take you on a journey of chocolatey bliss that will leave you enchanted.

Ingredients:

- 1 cup dairy-free chocolate chips (semi-sweet or dark)

- 1/2 cup canned full-fat coconut milk (shake the can well before opening)

Instructions:

1. In a heatproof bowl, add the dairy-free chocolate chips.

2. In a small saucepan, heat the coconut milk over medium heat

until it starts to simmer. Be careful not to let it boil.

3. Once the coconut milk is hot, pour it over the chocolate chips in the bowl.

4. Let the mixture sit for a minute or two to allow the heat from the coconut milk to melt the chocolate.

5. After a couple of minutes, gently stir the chocolate and coconut milk together until you achieve a smooth and glossy ganache.

6. If there are still some chocolate chips that haven't melted, you can place the bowl over a pot of simmering water (double boiler) and stir until everything is fully melted and combined.

7. Let the Vegan Chocolate Ganache cool slightly before using it as a glaze, dip, or drizzle for your favorite desserts.

Note: If the ganache is too thick after cooling, you can reheat it slightly to achieve the desired consistency.

9.3 Lemon Glaze with Stevia

At the heart of this glaze lies the pure zest of lemons, capturing the essence of sunny days and the brightness of nature's citrus bounty.

To achieve the perfect level of sweetness without sugar, we employ stevia, a plant-based sweetener that adds natural sweetness without affecting blood sugar levels.

The result is a glossy and vibrant Lemon Glaze that pairs exceptionally well with cakes, muffins, scones, and any dessert in need of a tangy and refreshing finish.

Our Lemon Glaze with Stevia is the epitome of a health-conscious indulgence, offering a guilt-free option for those seeking to reduce their sugar intake or manage diabetes while savoring the delectable tang of lemons.

Serve this glaze generously over your favorite desserts or drizzle it over fresh fruit for an invigorating treat that will awaken your taste buds.

Ingredients:

- 1 cup powdered stevia or stevia blend (adjust to taste)
- 2 tablespoons fresh lemon juice
- 1 tablespoon lemon zest
- 1-2 tablespoons water (as needed for desired consistency)

Instructions:

1. In a mixing bowl, whisk together the powdered stevia, fresh lemon juice, and lemon zest until well combined.

2. Add water, one tablespoon at a time, until you achieve the desired consistency. The glaze should be smooth and drizzle easily.

3. Taste the glaze and adjust the sweetness or tartness by adding more powdered stevia or lemon juice, according to your preference.

4. Once the Lemon Glaze with Stevia reaches your desired texture and sweetness, it is ready to use.

5. Drizzle the glaze generously over your favorite desserts, such as cakes, muffins, scones, or fruit, and let it set for a few minutes before serving.

Note: The glaze will slightly thicken as it sets, so adjust the consistency accordingly.

CONCLUSION

Throughout this cookbook, we've explored a diverse array of cake recipes that cater to individuals managing diabetes or those simply seeking wholesome and delicious options.

From flourless creations that celebrate the richness of ingredients like avocados, to low-sugar sponge cakes that reimagine classic favorites, and from nutritious fruit-based cakes that showcase the vibrancy of nature's bounty, to chocolate delights that prove you can have your cake and eat it too—each recipe has been thoughtfully crafted to bring joy to your kitchen and delight to your palate.

As you embark on your own baking adventures, whether it's for personal enjoyment, sharing with loved ones, or marking special occasions, we encourage you to approach each recipe with curiosity and creativity. Adapt the ingredients to suit your preferences, experiment with flavors, and don't hesitate to make each recipe your own.

Remember, these recipes are a starting point—an invitation to explore the fusion of ingredients, techniques, and tastes that culminate in a delightful masterpiece. Your journey doesn't end here; it continues with every cake you bake, every slice you share, and every smile you create.

Thank you for joining us on this flavorful expedition through "Diabetic Cake Recipes UK." We hope that this cookbook has empowered you to celebrate the joy of baking while embracing health-conscious choices, and that these recipes continue to be a source of inspiration in your culinary endeavors. May your kitchen always be filled with the warm aroma of freshly baked cakes and the sweet satisfaction of sharing your creations with those you cherish.